How to Eliminate Heart Burn and Acid Reflux Naturally

by M. Usman

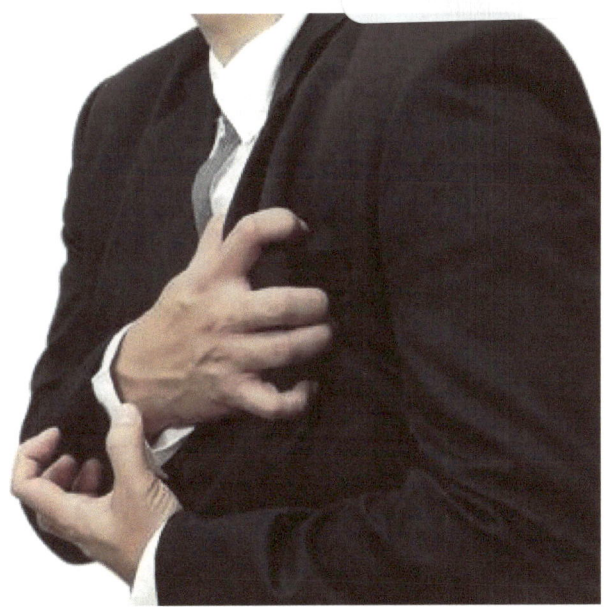

Health Learning Series

Mendon Cottage Books

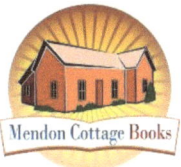

JD-Biz Publishing

Our books are available at

1. Amazon.com

2. Barnes and Noble

3. Itunes

4. Kobo

5. Smashwords

6. Google Play Books

Table of Contents

Introduction

Are you clueless how to get rid of heart burn? Do you need help overcoming the burning pain you experience before or after eating your meals? Is heart burn ruining your life? No matter how old your problem of heart burn may be, "How to get rid of heart burn and Acid Reflux Naturally" gives you a quick review of all homemade, herbal, allopathic and surgical remedies for heart burn.

Each chapter of this book gives you a deep insight to the basic causes of heart burn and helps answer your basic question "How to get rid of this condition?"

Following the guidelines regarding life style changes, eating habits and medical care, mentioned in this book, you can overcome this problem in a quick and effective manner and can prevent the relapse of symptoms.

Section one : What is heart burn?

"Heart burn" is a commonly used term for clinical condition known as "cardialgia", "pyrosis", "acid indigestion" or "acid reflux". It is a pain of radiating nature felt just behind the chest bone or epigatrium i.e. the upper central part of abdominal cavity. Sometimes the pain is also felt in the jaw or the back of body.

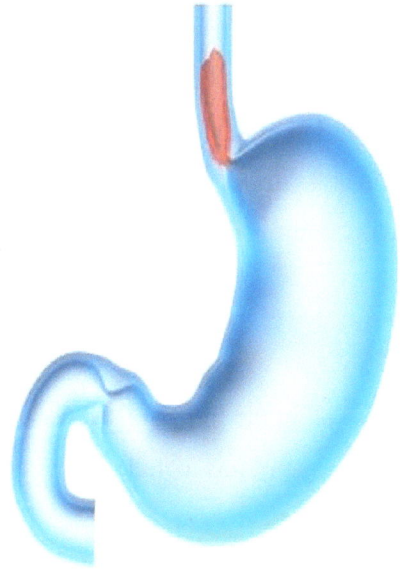

Human stomach is mainly concerned with the digestion of protein content of food. For this purpose, stomach produces an acidic "gastric juice". The "Lower esophageal sphincter" (LES) present at the junction of esophagus i.e. the tube that takes ingested food to the stomach, and stomach usually closely tightly during digestion of food and prevents the reflux of acidic contents of stomach back into the esophagus.

However, the functioning of lower esophageal sphincter (LES) is impaired due to any disease, trauma or congenital causes. In such conditions the sphincter can't close properly during the digestion of food. The raised intra gastric pressure forces the acidic contents of stomach to go back into the esophagus. These acidic contents, in turn, cause intense irritation of walls of esophagus which is then felt as a feeling of burning pain in the chest or upper abdominal region.

The mucosa i.e. lining, of lower end of esophagus can tolerate the abuse of this acidic reflux. But, repeated exposure to the acidic reflux from stomach causes the ulceration of mucosa and it leads to the repetition of symptoms of chest pain and burning with every meal intake. In this way, the eating habits are severely disturbed so is the quality of life.

Symptoms of heart burn

Heart burn presents itself in the form of variety of symptoms that vary in adults and children. These symptoms include:

- In adults.

    The most common symptoms of heat burn in adults include:
    - ➤ Dysphagia i.e. difficulty in swallowing.
    - ➤ Loss of appetite.
    - ➤ Nausea
    - ➤ Vomiting.

- ➢ Esophageal ulcerations and bleeding.
- ➢ Weight loss due to improper digestion of food and intense vomiting.

In children:

The most important symptoms in children include:

- ➢ The child feels nauseated and vomits repeatedly.
- ➢ The intensity and frequency of vomiting increases after feeding.
- ➢ The child cries and feels very uncomfortable.
- ➢ Frequent drooling of saliva.
- ➢ Decreased appetite.
- ➢ Significant loss of body weight.
- ➢ The child refuses to eat even when he is hungry.
- ➢ Choking due to blockade of air way if the regurgitated content of stomach makes way into the respiratory track.
- ➢ Wheezing and coughing.
- ➢ An unpleasant breath.

What are the causes of heart burn?

Any factor that alters the normal functioning of lower esophageal sphincter or leads to the increase in production of gastric juice can cause heart burn. All such causes can be divided into two basic groups:

- • Physiological causes.
- • Pathological causes.

Physiological causes of heart burn.

Physiological factors include all those natural processes that can develop symptoms of heart burn by altering body physiology or biochemistry. Such factors include:

Pregnancy:

During pregnancy, the female body undergoes immense physical and hormonal changes. The size of uterus increases in order to accommodate the increasing size of fetus. This over sized uterus pushes against the contents of abdomen. All other abdominal organs, including kidney and liver, are rigid and they are not compressed by the uterus. Stomach and intestines, being compressible, receive the insult of increasing size of uterus. The stomach is compressed and intra gastric pressure rises. This raised intra gastric pressure, in turn, causes the regurgitation of stomach contents into the esophagus causing heart burn.

The levels "progesterone" increase several folds during pregnancy. Progesterone relaxes the muscles of female body. The muscles of lower esophageal sphincter are also relaxed and the sphincter can't close properly while digestion leading to the reflux of acidic contents.

Food stuff:

Different types of food stuff can also cause heart burn. Such food stuff includes:

o   Caffeine: It is the major constituent of coffee, chocolates and carbonated beverages. It causes heart burn by increasing the production of stomach acid.

o   Alcohol: Increased alcohol intake causes heart burn by increasing the production of gastrin i.e. a stomach hormone, which in turn increases the production of stomach acid (HCl).

o   Oily food: Junk food, rich in oil, promotes the relaxation of lower esophageal sphincter and causes reflux of acidic contents.

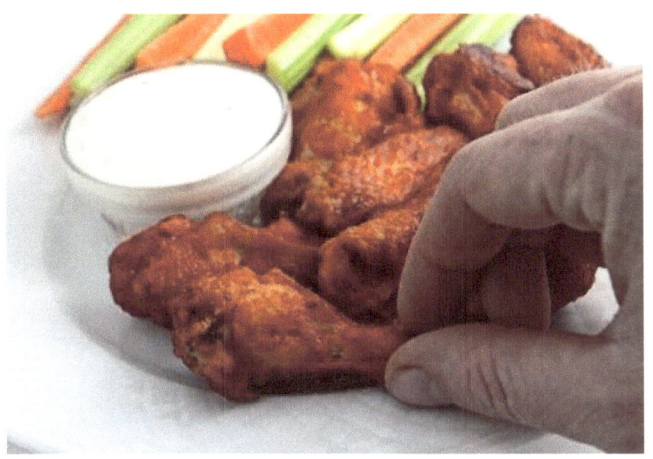

o   Spicy food: Spicy food strongly stimulates the production of stomach acid.

o   Over eating: Taking heavy meals or lying down immediately after food intake puts a lot of pressure against esophageal sphincter causing reflux.

o   Citrus juices: Citrus juices are another important cause of hear burn.

o   High protein diet: Stomach is meant to digest the production of protein in diet. More protein we take in our diet more is the production of gastric juice. This increased production of gastric juice in turn causes reflux and heart burn.

Pathological cause of heart burn:

Pathological causes of heart burn include all congenital deformities in body physiology and biochemistry, any disease or trauma that either disturbs the function of esophageal sphincter or increases the production of gastric juice. These pathological causes include:

Abnormal anti-reflux barrier:

Nature has provided our body with a barrier that prevents the reflux of acidic contents of stomach. The basic components of this barrier include lower esophageal sphincter, length of esophagus and curves of esophagus. In several congenital anomalies, the length of esophagus is less than usual. In other conditions, the normal curves of esophagus are absent. Such factors obliterate the anti-reflux barrier and it becomes easy for stomach contents to move into the esophagus.

Decreased emptying of stomach:

After the digestion of food, the pyloric sphincter relaxes allowing the "acidic chyme" to move from the stomach into the duodenum. However, any hormonal or motor abnormality that inhibits this activity of stomach can cause heart burn. Such factors include:

> ➢ Decreased parasympathetic impulses to the pyloric sphincter.
> ➢ Increased sympathetic impulses to the sphincter.
> ➢ Decreased production of "gastrin".
> ➢ Increased production of "cholysystokinin" i.e. gut hormone that inhibits gastric emptying.

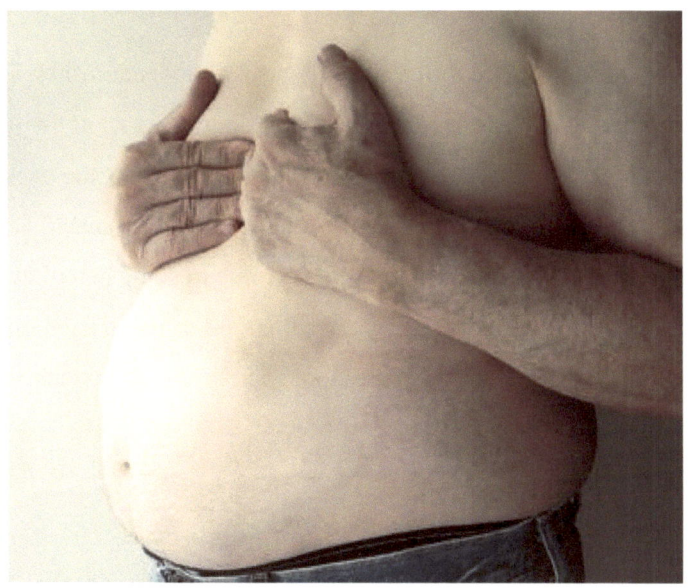

- ➢ Decreased production of "motilin" which causes the movements of stomach sluggish.
- ➢ Increased acidity of chyme entering into the duodenum also inhibits gastric emptying.
- ➢ Diabetes linked hyperglycemia also inhibits gastric emptying.

Obesity:

Most of the obese people complain of heart burn. The major cause of which is the increased amount of fat that gets deposited around the waist and abdomen. This extra fat compresses the content of abdomen, mainly the stomach. This raised intra-abdominal pressure leads to the improper functioning of esophageal sphincter causing heart burn.

Duodenal-gastric reflux:

This reflux is quite different form gastro-duodenal reflux. There is another sphincter called "pyloric sphincter" present at the junction of stomach and duodenum. This sphincter prevents the back movement of contents from duodenum into the stomach. However, due to some surgical complication or due to some hereditary causes, the sphincter weakens and allows the food to move from duodenum into the stomach. It raises the intra gastric pressure which in turn causes heart burn.

Post operative complications:

Vagus nerve it the major nerve that stimulate the motility of gut. In "vagotomy" the vagus nerve is cut surgically. As the result, the stimulatory impulses to the gut decrease and gastric emptying is delayed. The food remains in stomach for a long period of time and increases the intra gastric pressure. This raises intra gastric pressure in turn causes acid reflux and heart burn.

Hiatal hernias:

Esophagus makes way from the chest cavity into the abdominal cavity through a "hiatus" (opening) present in the diaphragm i.e. the muscular partition present between abdominal and chest cavity. In some cases the opening is larger than usual or the length of esophagus is lesser than usual. This causes the retraction of stomach from abdomen through that opening into the chest cavity. This raises the pressure inside the stomach and causes the regurgitation of food into the esophagus causing intense irritation and burning sensation in the chest region.

Zollinger Edison syndrome:

This is a congenital anomaly characterized by increased production of gastrin. This increased production of gastrin, in turn, increases the production of stomach acid that leads to reflux and heart burn.

Hypercalcimia:

This is a disorder characterized by increased production of serum calcium. High level of calcium strongly stimulates the production of gastric juice and high levels of gastric juices increases the chances of acid reflux and heart burn.

Section two: How to get rid of heart burn?

Heart burn is a common problem faced by a lot of people. That's why a lot of effort has been put in finding the causes and cures of this condition. Heart burn is a chronic condition that affects all the aspects of a person's life. It disturbs his eating habits and makes him feel uncomfortable all the times. The pain associated with heart burn makes it difficult for the person to perform his routine activities in an effective manner. Other symptoms like bad breath make it difficult for the person to socialize and sometimes put him in an embarrassing situation before his friends and family. Moreover, if the condition goes untreated it aggravates the damage done to esophagus and can cause serious complications like cancer of esophagus.

Luckily, there are a lot of ways in which heart burn can be treated. All the treatments benefit the person by providing a relief from this situation and improving the quality of life. In this section all the available treatments are discussed in detail. The basic treatments for heart burn include:

o   Life style changes.
o   Home remedies for heart burn.
o   Herbal treatment for heart burn.
o   Eating habits during heart burn.
o   Medication for heart burn.
o   Posture changes while sleeping.
o   Posture changes while eating.
o   Stress management and heart burn.
o   Surgical treatment for heart burn.

Life style changes

In most of the cases, the basic cause of heart burn is an inappropriate life style. Most of the people have got a stagnant life style. They haven't got enough time to go out for an exercise. This lack of physical activities makes a person prone to several health complications; heart burn is one of such complications. Minor changes in life style can bring about major changes in the physical and mental health of person. If someone has got heart burn, he should adopt following life style changes:

Small meals:
Whenever you eat, try to take small meals instead of heavy meals. Heavy meals cause heart burn is two ways:
- o By causing excessive distension of stomach. This distention puts a lot of pressure on LES and causes its relaxation.
- o Heavy meals trigger the production of large amount of acid in stomach.

Both these causes increase the reflux of acidic contents to the esophagus and develop symptoms of heart burn. So, avoid taking heavy meals. Take small meals instead.

No meal before bed:
Meals should strictly be avoided before going to bed. The activity of body muscle decrease significantly during sleep and they are relaxed. The relaxation of gut sphincters causes the reflux of food. Moreover, heavy meals before bed increase the production of gastric acid during sleep. Try not to eat anything for at least 2-3 hours before going to

bed. This gap is necessary because it allows the stomach and intestines to digest the food properly and thus reflux is significantly reduced.

Avoid lying down after meals:

Most of the people are in the habit of lying down immediately after meals. This is one of the major causes of heart burn in majority of population. When a person lies down after meals, the pressure on LES increases and the distended stomach pushes the sphincter to an open position. So, a minor habit of not lying down immediately after meal can make a big difference in heart burn situation.

Eat slowly:

Most of the people that are in the habit of eating very fast complain of heart burn after meals. This habit causes acid reflux because of two reasons:

o   When you eat rapidly, the stomach doesn't get enough time to digest the food in an effective manner. So, the stomach tries to improve digestion by increasing the production of acid.

o   When the space of the stomach is rapidly filled with food, the air doesn't get enough time to escape. The entrapped air increases the intra-gastric pressure leading to the reflux of acidic contents.

So, following things should be kept in mind while eating:

o   Try to eat slowly.

- Chew your food properly before swallowing.
- Try to eat food in small bits.

Lose extra fat:

Nature has designed human body, and all of its systems, to conserve extra calories we eat in the form of fat. So, whenever we eat more than the requirements of our body it stores the excess calories in the form of fat in areas like around waist, hips and chest. When the fats deposits around the stomach increase, they start to put a lot of pressure on abdominal contents especially the stomach. So, obesity is the basic culprit of heart burn in most of the cases. Try to lose your weight by following few guidelines:

- Exercise regularly as exercise speed up the consumption of extra fat.
- Eat protein rich diet, high in fibers.
- Avoid eating junk food rich in saturated fat and cholesterol.
- Avoid over eating.

Sit in upright posture after meals:

Try to sit in upright posture for at least 30-45 minutes after each meal. Sitting in an upright posture helps speed up the emptying of stomach and prevents its distention.

Walk after meal:

Don't walk immediately after meals. Instead, walk after 30-45 minutes. A small walk helps speed up the digestion of your food and emptying of stomach.

Avoid exercise after meals:

Avoid heavy exercises for at least one hour after the meals. Heavy exercises cause heart burn in two ways:

- o Heavy exercise after meals cause increase in tension of muscles, including the abdominal muscles. So, these tensed muscles put a lot of pressure on stomach.
- o Exercise increases the sympathetic drive of body. This causes the relaxation of LES.

Avoid tight clothing:

Sometimes, the cause of heart burn can be as simple as tight clothing. Clothing having tight waists would definitely put a lot of pressure on your stomach. Try to wear loose clothes that feel comfortable.

Eat healthy diet:

A proper and healthy diet plan can help in decreasing the symptoms associated with heart burn. Make sure your diet plan has following features:

- o Eat vegetables and fruits instead of meat and pork.
- o Eat food stuff that is rich in fibers.

- o Avoid oily food.
- o Avoid spicy food.
- o Avoid carbonated beverages.
- o Avoid use of animal oils while cooking. Use plant oils like olive oil.
- o Try to eat homemade food that is cooked hygienically.

Home remedies for heart burn

Several home remedies are available for heart burn. All such remedies are simple and inexpensive, yet very effective in the cure of heart burn. All these home remedies come straight from your cup board or refrigerator. Different home remedies for heart burn include:

Chew gum:

Chewing gum increases the production of saliva in mouth. Saliva is alkaline because of the production of bicarbonate ions. These bicarbonate ions help neutralize the acid produced by stomach.

Apple cider vinegar:

It is an effective home remedy for heart burn. You can make it at home but both tablet and liquid forms are available in stores. It helps in the digestion of food and induces a soothing effect during the periods of heart burn. The liquid preparations should be diluted properly in water before use.

Ginger:

It is one of the most effective home remedies available for heart burn. Ginger has got an excellent anti-inflammatory effect thus it prevents the inflammation caused by heart burn. Moreover, it provides a soothing effect and helps reduce the pain associated with heart burn. You can add ginger in your tea or can use it in your daily food.

Baking soda:

Add ½ tea spoon of baking soda in a cup of water and mix it well. Drink this mixture after meals. Baking soda is alkaline in nature so it helps neutralize the acid produced by the stomach. However, the use of this preparation should be avoided by the patients with high blood pressure as baking soda contains significant amount of sodium and sodium causes water retention and increase in blood pressure.

Garlic:

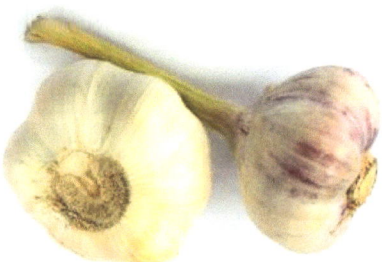

Garlic is another important home remedy available for heart burn. It has got strong anti-septic effects that can help cure the infection and heart burn caused by H.pylori infections.

Glutamine rich food:

Eat glutamine rich food as it has got strong anti-inflammatory properties. Glutamine is mainly present in:

- Fish
- Spinach
- Egg

Turmeric:

Turmeric helps cure heart burn in two ways:

- It speed up the digestion process going on in the stomach thus prevents the accumulation of food in the stomach and building of intra-gastric pressure.
- It has got excellent healing properties so it helps rebuild the mucosa of esophagus damaged during the periods of acid reflux.

Honey:

It is one of the most effective home remedies for heart burn. It has got extreme soothing and anti-inflammatory effects. Add honey in your drinks and foods.

Digestive enzyme supplements:

Take digestive enzyme supplements, like bromaline, easily available in market. These supplements help speed up the digestion process of stomach thus helps reduce the production of acid.

Herbal treatment for heart burn.

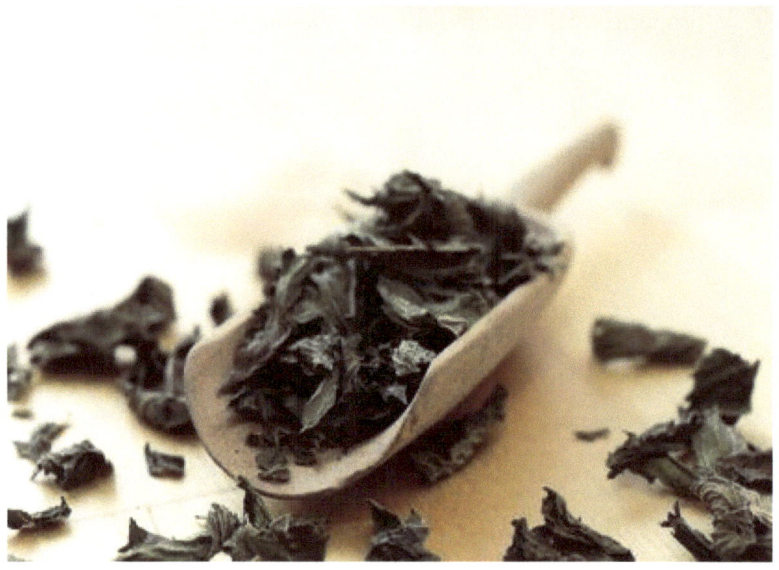

A lot of herbs are being used for the treatment of heart burn for long period of time. All these remedies provide a natural cure for heart burn. Use of herbs has got no side effects and these herbs can be used by almost all the people. Unlike the medicines, use of herbs is quite inexpensive and doesn't require any expertise. The effectiveness of these herbs is universally recognized and herbal method of treatment is still being widely practiced in a lot of countries of world. Different herbs used for the cure of heart burn include:

Licorice:

Herbal licorice is effective in patients with chronic heart burn. It forms a protective layer around the mucosa of stomach and esophagus thus prevents the erosion of this mucosa caused by stomach acid. However, several complain were reported by hypertensive patients that use if licorice further increases their blood pressure. So, the use of herbal licorice is not recommended in hypertensive patients.

Aloe Vera extracts:

It is one of the most effective herbal remedies available for heart burn. These extracts are easily available in tablet or liquid form. Aloe Vera helps cure heart burn in following manner:

- o It forms a protective covering around the mucosa of stomach and esophagus thus limits the damaged produced by the acidic contents of stomach.
- o It helps suppress the production of stomach acid, one of the basic causes of heart burn.
- o It has got anti-inflammatory effects thus helps cure the damage caused by acidic reflux.
- o It has a soothing affect when used during periods of pain associated with heart burn.

Basal leaves:

Chewing basal leaves help neutralize the acidity of stomach. It has soothing effects and helps cure bad breath.

Herbal barberry:

Eating 200-500 mg of herbal barberries in a day helps fight heart burn due to its following affects:

- o It helps the digestion of food thus prevents distention of stomach.
- o It promotes the relaxation of stomach muscles. Relaxations of these muscles decrease the chances of reflux.

Fennel tea:

It's an herbal tea that has got following affects:

- o It causes relaxation of stomach muscles.
- o It promotes the food digestion.
- o It's very rich in glycine, an amino acid that suppresses the release of gastric juice.

Chamomile tea:

It's a commonly used herbal remedy for heart burn. It helps reduce heart burn in three ways:

- o It helps neutralize the acidic contents of stomach thus prevents the damage caused by acid.
- o It improves the functioning of LES.
- o It has got potent anti-bacterial effects thus help cure heart burn in the cases of bacterial infections.

Both these factors prevent the reflux of acid into the esophagus and provide an effective relief from heart burn.

Slippery elm:

It's an herb that neutralizes the excess stomach acid spreads mucilage like covering over the stomach mucosa.

Marshmallow:

It's an herb that has anti-inflammatory and protective effects on stomach and esophageal mucosa. Drinking marshmallow tea for 2-3 times a day helps in the cure of heart burn.

Lemon balm:

Lemon balm is herbal in nature is derived from a plant with lemon like scent. It has got strong anti-bacterial and anti-viral effects. It's used when a person complains of nausea, vomiting, heart burn and flatulence.

Eating habits during heart burn.

The functioning of stomach is directly related with the food we eat. A lot of food stuff triggers the production of stomach acids, while others improve the functioning of stomach. So, minor changes in eating habits bring about major changes. The food groups can be widely divided into two groups:

- Triggers foods.
- Foods that help relieve heart burn.

Trigger foods:

A number of food stuff strongly triggers the production of stomach acid thus greatly aggravate the situation in heart burn. So, the use of such food stuff should be strictly avoided. Such food includes:

Oily food:

Oily food aggravates heart burn because of following basic reasons:

- o Oily food, like French fires and fried chicken pieces, require a long time to digest. So, such food remains in stomach for a longer period of time and stimulates the secretion of gastric juice.
- o Secondly, oily food makes the movements of stomach sluggish. So, the emptying of stomach is delayed and intra-gastric pressure starts to rise. This increase in intra-gastric pressure, in turn, promotes acid reflux.

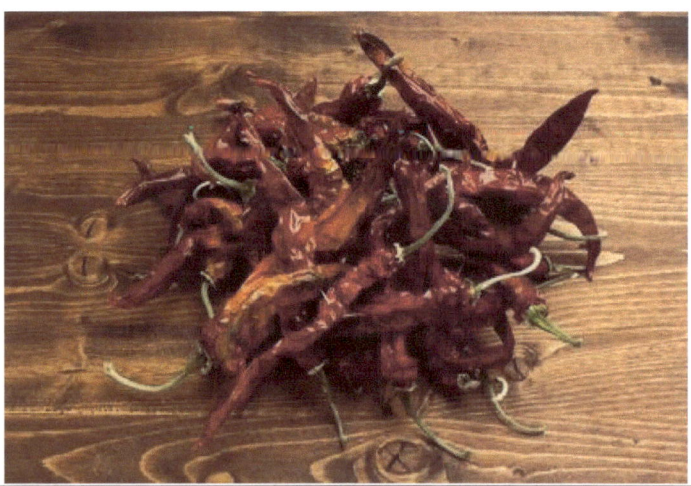

Spicy food:

Spicy food is another trigger of heart burn. Spices present in food irritate the stomach and cause it to secrete more HCl. Moreover, spices promote the damage of mucosa.

Meat :

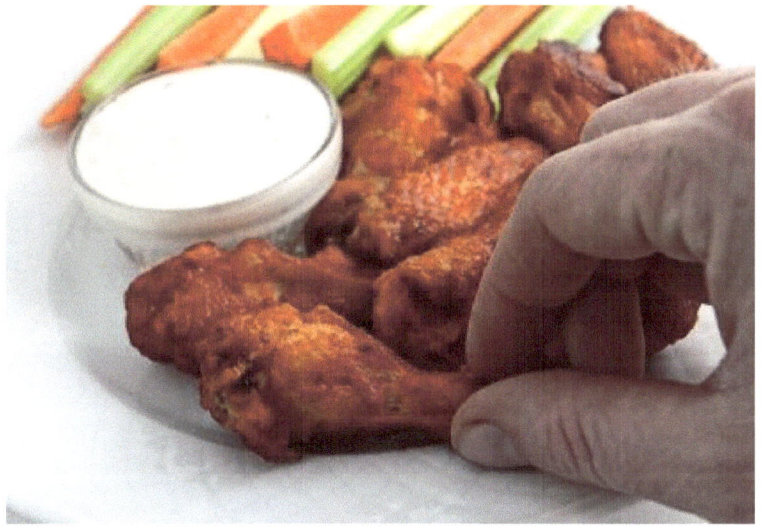

Stomach is mainly meant to digest the protein contents of food. All the meat products, including chicken, pork, beef, meat, sausages, hot dogs etc, are very rich in protein contents. The presence of protein in stomach strongly stimulates the production of stomach acid so that the proteins can be digested in an effective manner. So, the over use of protein diet should be avoided in heart burn.

Carbonated drinks:

The use of carbonated drinks should be avoided during heart burn because these beverages not only decrease the pH of stomach but also promote the secretion of HCl.

Dairy products:

The dairy products, like cheese, butter, milk, cream and shakes, should be avoided in heart burn because these products are extremely rich in calcium and calcium is a strong trigger for gastric juice secretion.

Caffeine:

It's mainly present in coffee, tea and chocolates. Caffeine is a strong trigger of gastric juice release. So, the use of caffeine containing food should be limited in heart burn.

Gluten:

Some people show allergy to gluten present in grains by increasing the production of gastric juice. So, such people should eat gluten free food.

Alcohol:

Alcohol should be strictly avoided since it is a strong irritant.

Citrus juices:

Citrus juices make the pH of stomach acidic and irritate the stomach mucosa to increase the production of gastric juice. That's why use of citric juice, like orange juice, grape fruit juice etc, should be avoided in chronic heart burn.

Food to eat during heart burn.

A lot of food stuff helps in the normal function of stomach by increasing its motility, decreasing the production of acids and anti-inflammatory effects. Such food includes:

Fruits :

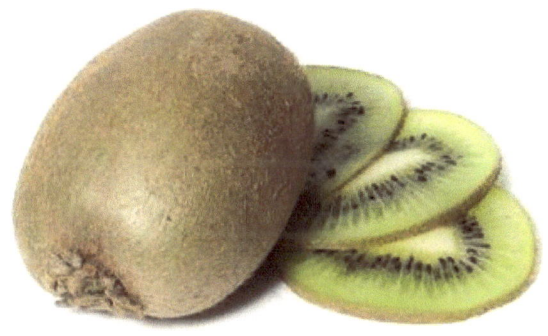

Several fruit, including kiwi fruit, peach, apricot, banana and melons, are advised during heart burn. All these fruits help in the reduction of heart burn because of two basic effects:

o These fruits are rich in fiber that increase the motility of stomach and increase the rate of its emptying.

o Moreover, these fruits help in the suppression of the secretion of stomach acids.

Fresh juices:

Drink fresh fruit juices. All the juices are rich in essential nutrients and help improve the activity of stomach. However, the use of citrus fruit juices should be avoided as they trigger the acid production.

Water:

Keep yourself adequately hydrated by drinking 8-10 glasses of water. Water promotes the normal movements of gut and helps neutralize the acidic contents of stomach.

Potassium rich food:

Potassium rich food such as sweet potatoes and apple cider vinegar is suggested in acid reflux. Potassium causes the contraction of the muscles of lower esophageal sphincter and prevents the back lash of food into the esophagus.

Vegetables:

Vegetables are highly recommended food during heart burn. This food group includes vegetables like carrot, spinach, cucumber, potatoes, ginger, garlic and all green leafy vegetables. Vegetables help reduce the stomach acidity due to following basic reasons:

- o Vegetables are highly rich in fibers that promote the movements of gut.
- o Raw vegetables are somewhat alkaline in nature that helps neutralize stomach acids.
- o Some vegetables contain certain enzymes that help in the digestion of food.

Whole grains:

Eat whole grains like oats, rice, bread and cereals to get rid of heart burn. These grains are highly rich in fibers. Fibers are rich in cellulose, a sugar that is not digested in humans. As the result the motility of gut is increased and the food is not allowed to stay into the stomach long enough to cause symptoms of heart burn.

Beans:

The patients of heart burn are strictly advised to avoid meat and meat products. But problem arises to find an alternative protein source since there is nothing as good as meat when it comes to protein. But, beans are an excellent substitute of meat that is rich in proteins. So, beans fulfill the protein requirements of body without increasing the production of acid.

Salad:

Add salads in your daily diet plan. Salads are rich in essential nutrients like proteins, minerals and vitamins. They are very rich in fibers also. They suppress hunger and decrease the production of stomach acid.

White meat:

White meat, like sea food, is safer to use as compared to red meat. It is rich in protein yet doesn't cause excessive release of acid.

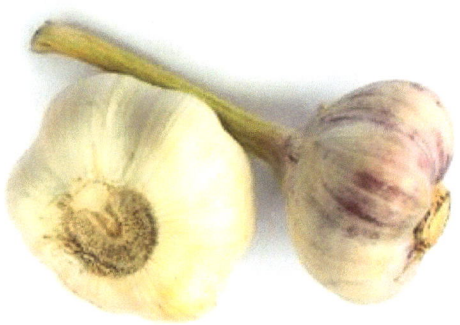

Garlic and ginger:

Add Ginger and garlic in your routine food as they have got excellent:

- o   Anti-bacterial properties
- o   Anti-viral properties.

o   Anti-inflammatory properties.

o   Ability to suppress acid production.

o   Soothing effect when used.

Oat meal:

Eating oat meal helps reduce the symptoms of heart burn.

Medicines for heart burn

A vast variety of medicines are available for the treatments of heart burn. All the medicines have got their own mechanism of action, route of administration, dose, effects, side effects and contra-indications. All these aspects of drugs for heart burn are studied in detail in the following section.

Anti-acids:

One of the basic causes of heart burn is the excessive production of stomach acid. When HCl is produced in excess, a burst of electrical impulses is sent to the brain and it is interpreted as pain in the chest and upper abdomen area. Anti-acids are alkaline drugs that help neutralize the acidic secretions produced by the stomach. This way the pain associated with heat burn is suppressed with use of anti-acids. The best anti-acids used for this purpose include:

o   Milk of magnesia.

o   Surpass gum.

o   Alka seltzer.

o   Alternagel.

o   Gaviscon.

o   Mylanta.

Active ingredients of anti-acids:

The active ingredients of anti-acids include:

o Calcium carbonate: It acts rapidly and helps increase the pH of stomach by neutralizing the acidic contents.

o Sodium carbonate: It is another active ingredient of anti-acids with action similar to calcium carbonate. But, its duration of action is lesser as compared to calcium carbonate.

o Aluminium hydroxide: It helps neutralize the acidic pH of stomach and makes a protective covering over the stomach preventing the action of acid on stomach mucosa.

o Magnesium trisilicate: It also helps neutralize stomach acids.

Indications for giving anti-acids:

These anti-acids are given in peptic ulcers, GERD and heart burn.

Contra-indications:

There are some conditions in which the use of anti-acids is not advised. Such conditions include:

o Anti-acids containing high levels of sodium are not given to patients with hypertension, cardiac or renal failure and pregnant women because it aggravates there condition by the retention of water and increase of blood pressure.

o Anti-acids with high levels of calcium may develop complications like alkalosis, kidney stones and hpercalcimia.

- Aluminum containing anti-acids may cause brain damage and thus should be avoided in patients with mental impairments.

Histamine 2 blockers :

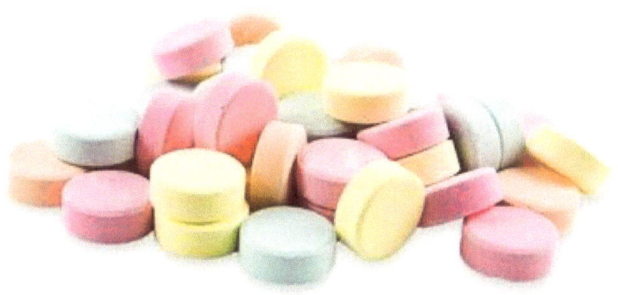

Histamine acts on histamine receptors present on stomach cells, which are responsible for the release of gastric juice. So, histamine is a potent stimulant of gastric juice release. These drugs help reduce the action of histamine on its receptors and the secretion of acid is decreased as a result. The most commonly use histamine 2 blockers include:

- Axid
- Pepcid
- Tagemet

- Conditions in which these drugs are given : These drugs are given in peptic and esophageal ulcer, GERD and heart burn.

- Common side effects : The most common side effects of these drugs include:
  - Nausea.
  - Vomiting.
  - Improper bowel movements.
  - Sexual dysfunction in males.
  - Decreased number of platelets and increased tendency to bleed.

- Proton pump inhibitors:

  These are energy dependent pumps present in the cells of gastric mucosa. These pumps actively transport Hydrogen ions into the lumen of stomach. These hydrogen ions combine with chloride ions and HCl is produced as a result. So, if the activity of this pump is blocked the formation of stomach acid can be decreased. The most important drugs of this group include:
  - Nexium
  - Prilosec
  - Prevacid
  - Aciphex

- Indications and contra-indications:

  The indications are same as all other heart burn medications.

  However, the important contra-indications for these drugs include:
  - Pregnant females.
  - Women breast feeding their children.
  - Patients with liver disease.

- side effects:

The common side effects of these medicines include:

- o Abdominal cramps.
- o Flatulence.
- o Nausea.
- o Vomiting.
- o Improper bowel movements.
- o Headaches.

Prokinetic drugs:

Another way to decrease the chances of acid reflux is to remove all the gastric contents as early as possible because when the food hoards up into the esophagus it increases the intra-gastric pressure and causes the reflux of food. Prokinetic drugs increase the motility of stomach and intestines. In this way the food is removed from the stomach before it can build up the intra-gastric pressure. The prototypes of this group include:

- o Benzamide.
- o Cisapride.
- o Metoclopromide.
- o Domperidone.

Indications:

The use of these drugs is recommended in conditions like:

- o Peptic ulcers.
- o Esophageal ulcers.

o   Heart burn.

o   Constipation.

o   Bloating.

o   Vomiting.

Side effects:

The most common side effects seen with the use of these drugs include:

o   Diarrhea.

o   Loss of weight.

o   Fatigue.

o   Feeling of restlessness.

o   Anxiety and nervousness.

Posture changes while sleeping.

Most of the people complain of heart burn while they are asleep. The basic culprit in most of such cases is improper sleeping posture that triggers a series of changes that result in the development of following events:

o   A wrong sleeping posture increases the production of acid in the stomach.

o   When a person lay down on his stomach the rate of stomach emptying is delayed.

o   The laying down on one's stomach increases the intra-gastric pressure further. This increased pressure causes the LES to open and regurgitation of food into the esophagus starts. This irritates the lining of esophagus and cause intense pain and burning sensation over the region of chest and upper abdomen.

o Sometimes, the intra-gastric pressure is increased to such an extent that the food makes way to the upper respiratory track. It causes blockade of respiration.

Here are some suggestions for the patients of heart burn to cure this condition by bring minor changes in their sleeping habits.

Sleep on your right side:

Sleeping on your right side helps reduce acid reflux in two ways:

o It decreases the pressure on stomach as compared to the people that are in the habit of sleeping on their left side.

o Sleeping on your right side promotes the empting of your stomach. This way food is not allowed to stay in the stomach long enough to increase the intra gastric pressure.

Don't sleep on your stomach:

It is a common finding that sleeping on one's stomach gives a burning pain in the chest and upper abdomen region. Such sleeping posture is inappropriate because it increases the intra-gastric pressure and promotes the reflux of acid. So sleeping in such posture should be avoided.

Keep your head elevated:

The patients with acid reflux are suggested to use pillow to keep their hear 5-6 inches above the level of rest of their body. In this posture, the level of esophagus becomes higher as compared to the stomach and the entry of acid into the esophagus stops due to the action of gravity.

Posture changes while eating.

A bad posture while eating can significantly increases the susceptibility of development of acid reflux and heart burn. Most of the people don't pay much attention to their sitting posture while eating and sit in an awkward position that increases the acid reflux. Something as simple as posture changes while eating can prevent the development of heartburn.

- ➢ Always eat when you are comfortably seated. Avoid eating while running, walking or lying down. Eating in such positions interferes with the digestion of food and promotes regurgitation of food. The gastric emptying is delayed and intra-gastric pressure rises. So, always try to sit down properly before you start eating.
- ➢ Try not to bend over the dining table while eating. It puts pressure over the stomach and causes back lash of food into the esophagus. Try to maintain an upright posture while eating on a dining table.
- ➢ Choose to sit on a comfortable chair that gives proper support to your back.
- ➢ Try to keep your knees and hips on the same level while sitting on the chair. It'll help gravity pull the food away from your esophagus.
- ➢ Keep your feet on the floor while eating.

> ➤ Avoid unnecessary movements while eating. Such movements hinder with the normal digestion of food.

Stress management and heart burn.

The people that face periods of chronic stress often complain of gastric reflux. Acid reflux further worsens their condition. Stress increases the sympathetic discharge inside the body, which, in turn, causes heart burn because of following basic reason:

> ➤ Sympathetic discharge decreases the flow of blood to the muscles of body but the supply of blood to the organs, like gut, is reduced. As the result, the movements of gut become sluggish and the rate of emptying decreases.
> ➤ Sympathetic discharge decreases the motility of gut by countering the intrinsic activity of enteric nervous system i.e. an integrative unit present in the walls of gut that controls the normal motility of gut and is stimulated by Para-sympathetic but is inhibited by sympathetic nervous system.
> ➤ Sympathetic discharges causes relaxation of LES.
> ➤ Stress causes an increase in the release of gastric juice.

These factors decrease the stomach motility and intra-gastric pressure increases. Moreover, the production of acid is increased. As the result, the reflux of highly acidic stomach contents starts during periods of intense stress.

How to manage stress?

Stress, and therefore heart burn, can be managed by simple life style changes. Such changes include:

- o Exercise regularly as it increases the supply of blood to brain and other parts of body and help decrease stress.
- o Try relaxing techniques like yoga.
- o Try relaxing muscle techniques.
- o Get adequate sleep and improve both the quality and quantity of sleep.
- o Spare some time for hobbies laid gardening or anything that pleases you.
- o Be active socially. Go in family gathering and go out with your friends.
- o Don't discuss those topics that increase your stress.
- o Don't try to burden yourself with work.
- o Add humor to your life.
- o Don't try to control the uncontrollable.
- o Understand your limits and try to act accordingly.
- o Consult a physician or a psychiatrist.

Surgical treatments for heart burn.

When all the other therapies fail, the last choice for the treatment of heart burn and acid reflux is the surgical correction of the problem. Surgery is considered when the patient is prone to development of one of following conditions:

- o Barrett's esophagus.

- Severe esophagitis.
- Carcinoma of esophagus.
- Constriction of esophagus.

Types of surgery:

Two types of surgical methods are used for the correction of acid reflux:

- Laparoscopy.
- Radio frequency therapy.

Laparoscopy:

In this procedure, a small hole is made in the walls of stomach and camera guided tube is inserted into the abdomen. A team of surgeons develop a new barrier between esophagus and stomach thus the chances of acid reflux are reduced to minimum. This procedure has got following basic advantages:

- The healing of wound is very quick.
- The chances of infection are less.
- Less dangerous as compared to open surgery.
- Takes less time to complete.

Radio frequency therapy:

It's a modern technique used for the treatment of heart burn. In this procedure, a high energy laser beam is thrown on the lower part of esophagus. It creates a fibrotic clot in that area of esophagus. As the result, the opening between stomach and esophagus is reduced in size and chances of reflux decrease as well. This method has got following advantages:

- No chances of infection.
- No bleeding.
- Body is not opened.
- Takes less time.
- Healing is complete and quick.

Photo credits:

All Images Licensed by Fotolia.com

Antacid Tablets

© *Steve Carroll - Fotolia.com*

Finger grabbing buffalo chicken wing

© *Cappi Thompson - Fotolia.com*

Heart attack of a businessman

© *Nolight - Fotolia.com*

Peperonciniessiccati

© *MarcoBagnoliElflaco - Fotolia.com*

Kiwi fruit isolated on white

© *MaksimŠmeljov - Fotolia.com*

Garlic

© *shreddhead - Fotolia.com*

Heavy man with pain in chest

© *nebari - Fotolia.com*

MagenmitmarkierterSpeiseröhre

© *Sebastian Kaulitzki - Fotolia.com*

Bio Minztee

© *cirquedesprit - Fotolia.com*

Author Bio

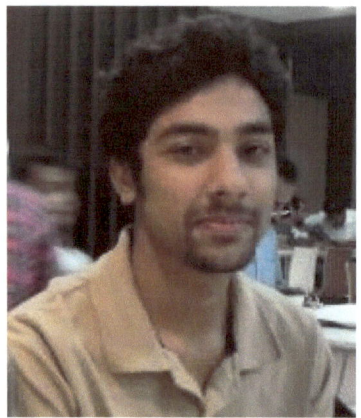

Muhammad Usman is a distinguished medical graduate of Allama iqbal medical college (AIMC). He is a professional writer who has been in the field for more than 4 years. During this time he has produced 10,000+ articles, blogs and eBooks on various niches related to diseases, health, fitness, nutrition and well-being. He is a regular contributor to several journals related to medicine and surgery. He is the editor of several journals and newspapers.

Check out some of the other JD-Biz Publishing books

[Gardening Series on Amazon]

Download Free Books!

http://MendonCottageBooks.com

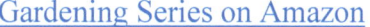

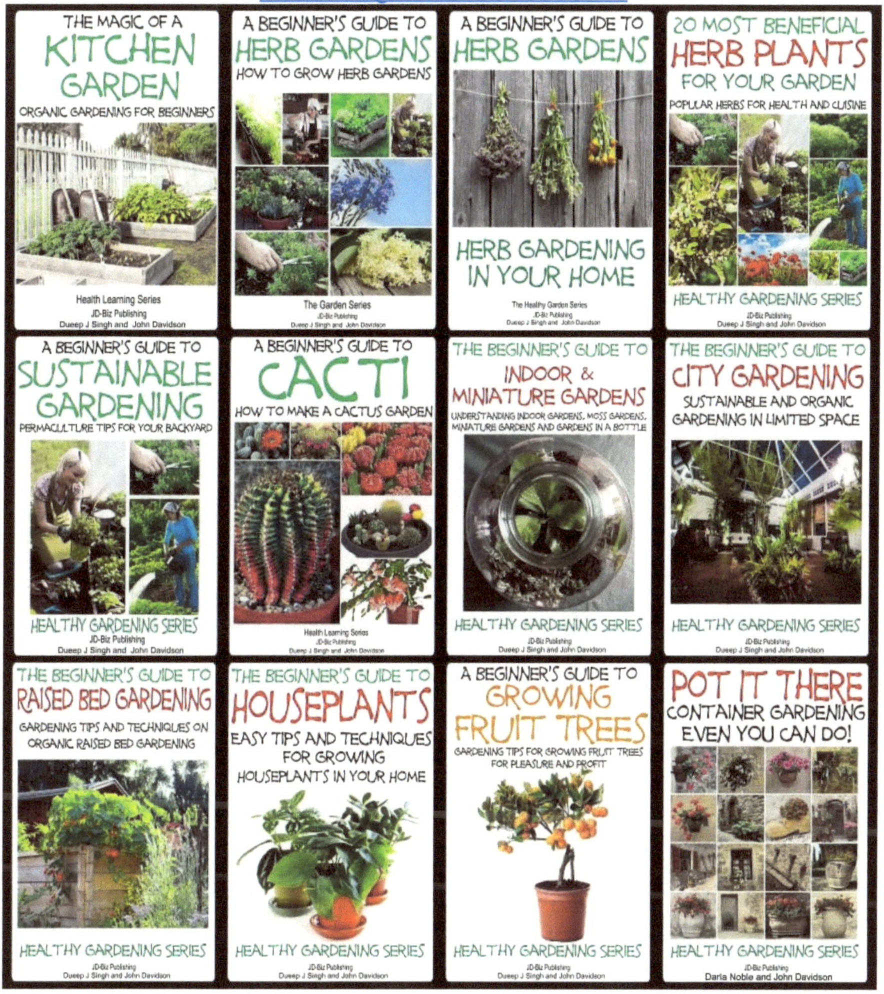

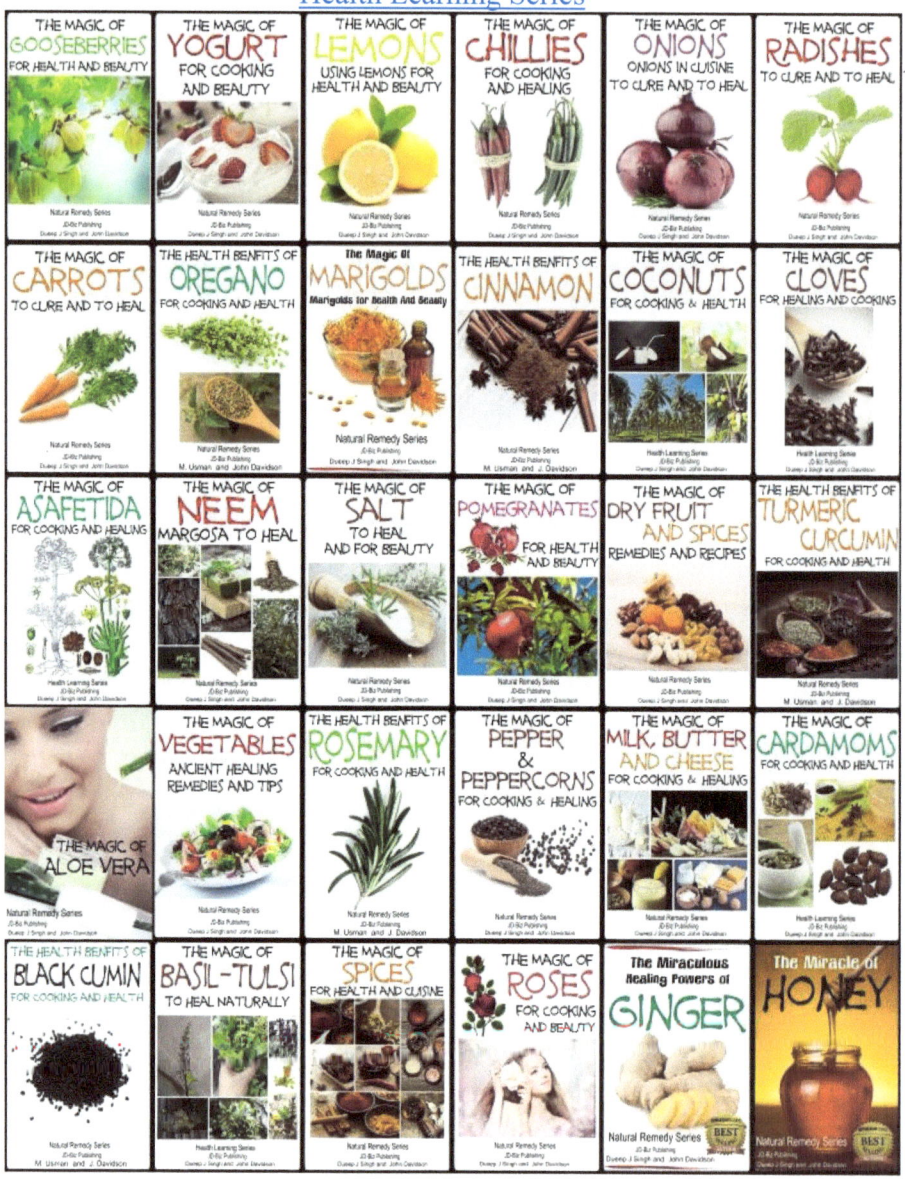

Country Life Books

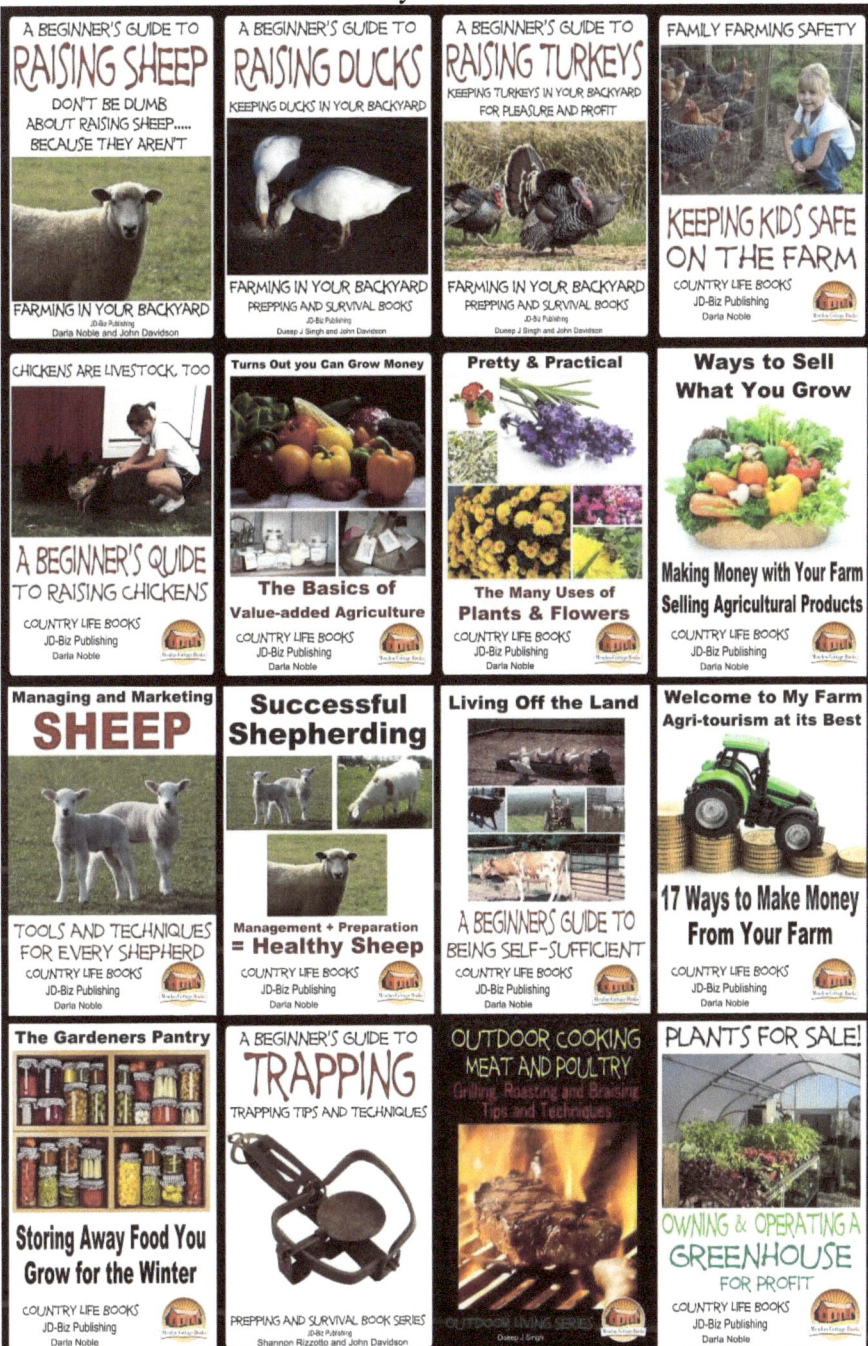

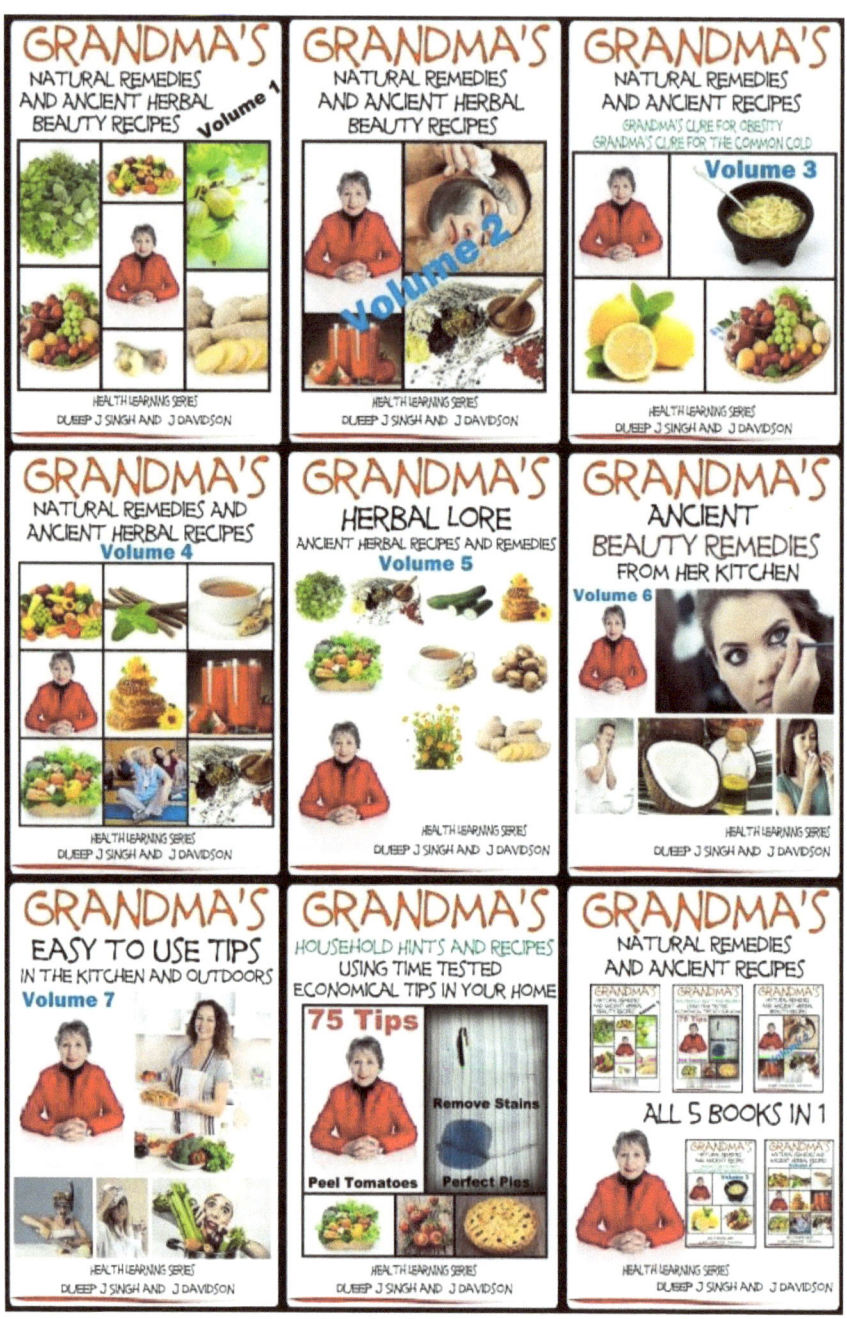

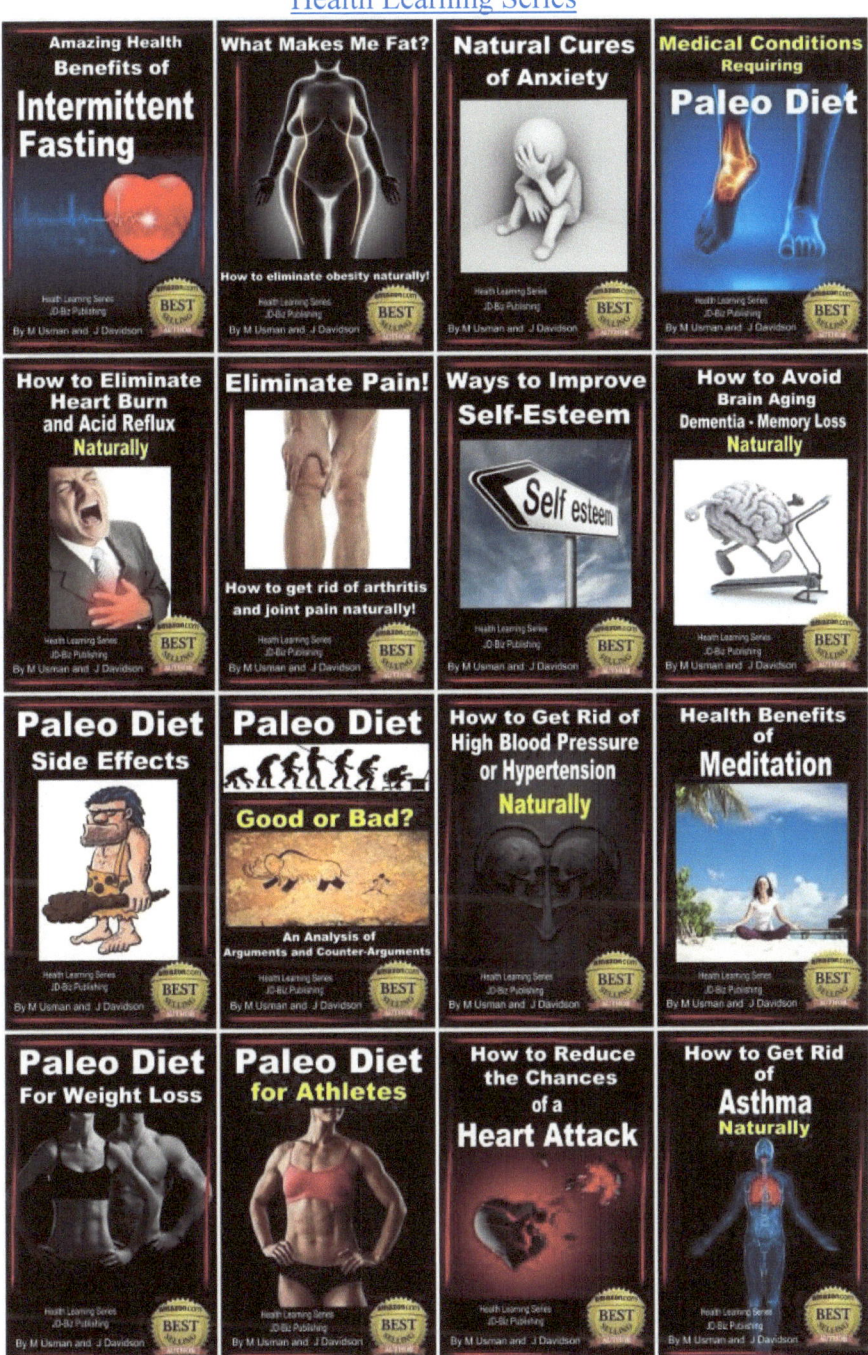

Amazing Animal Book Series

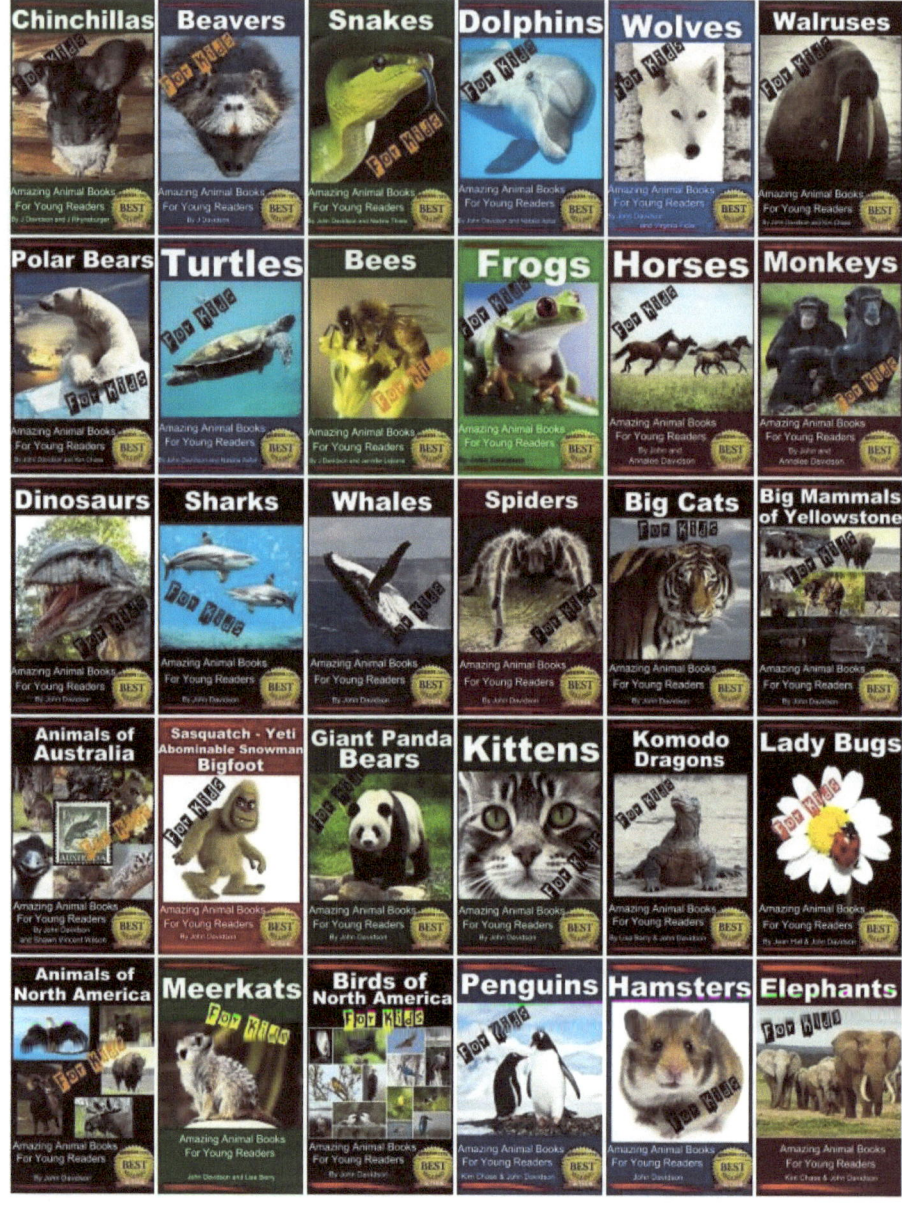

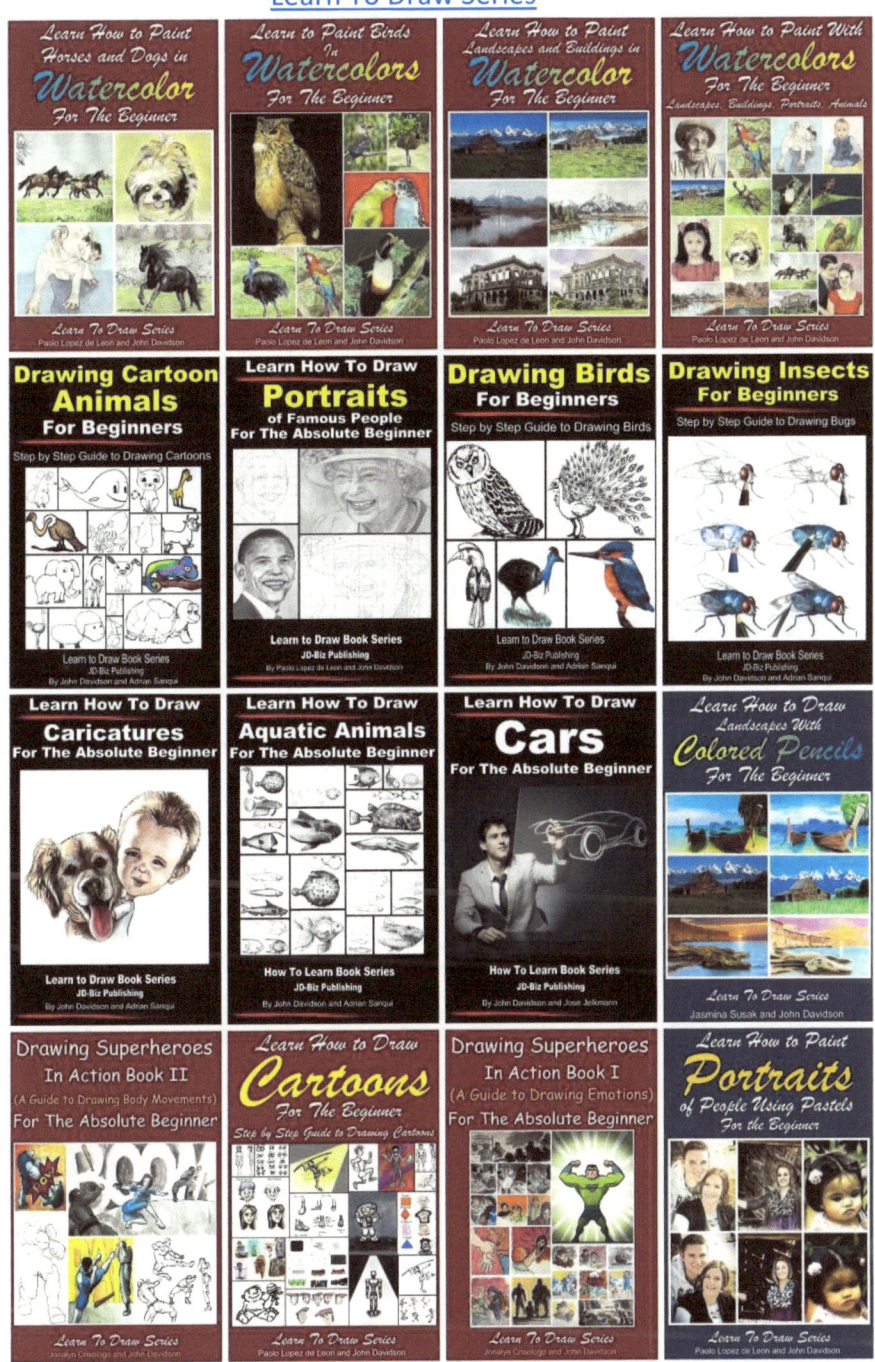

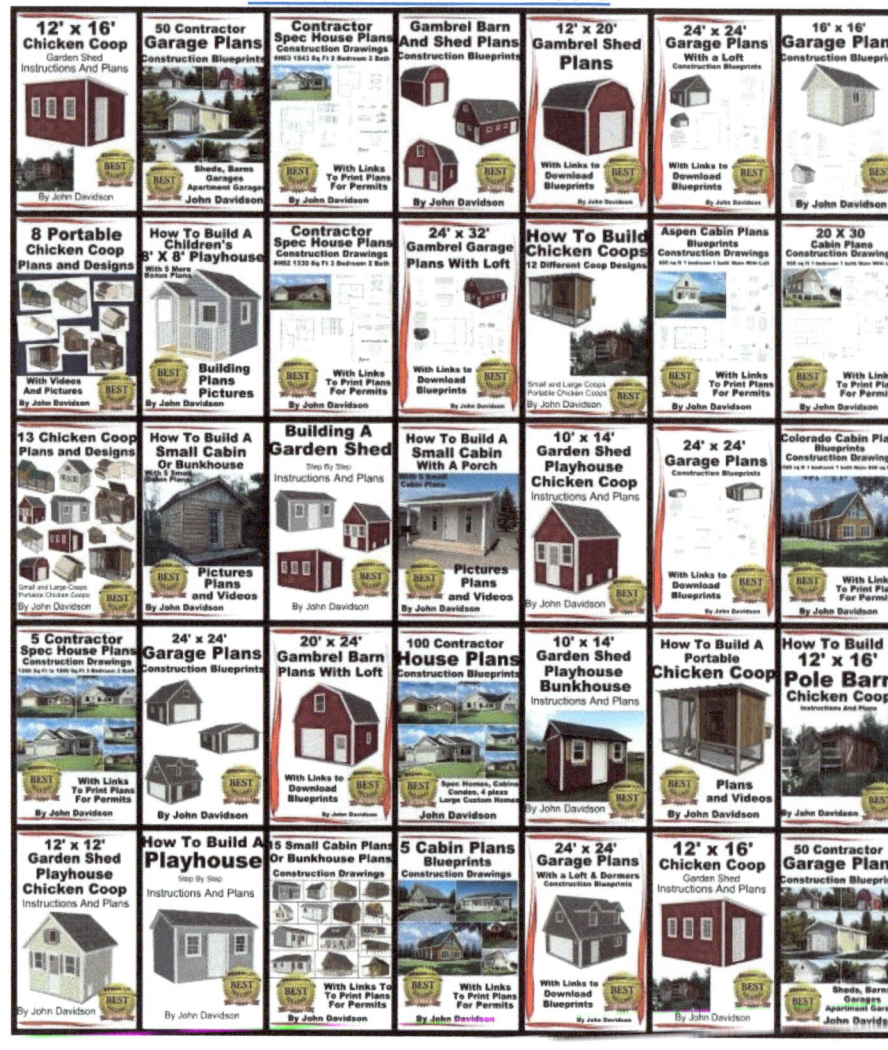

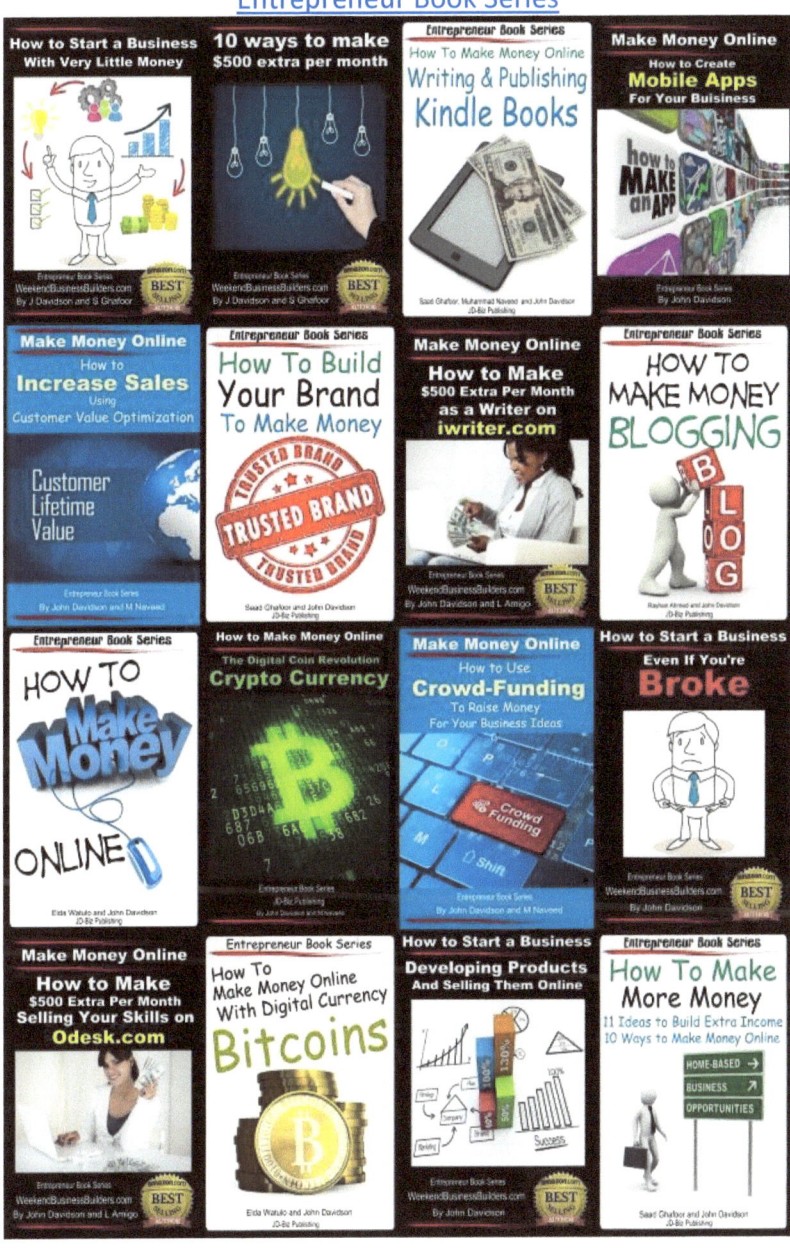

Our books are available at

1. Amazon.com
2. Barnes and Noble
3. Itunes
4. Kobo
5. Smashwords
6. Google Play Books

Download Free Books!
http://MendonCottageBooks.com

Publisher

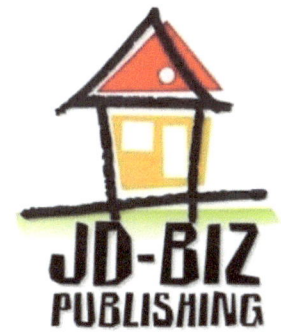

JD-Biz Corp

P O Box 374

Mendon, Utah 84325

http://www.jd-biz.com/

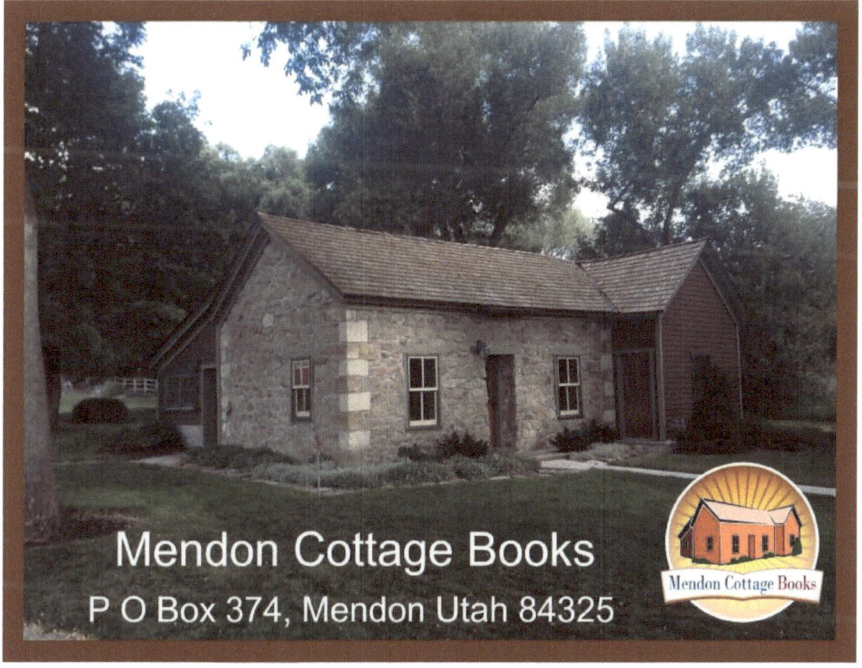

www.ingramcontent.com/pod-product-compliance
Lightning Source LLC
Chambersburg PA
CBHW050822290526
45792CB00001B/225